I DID IT!

Tummy Tuck Surgery – An Intimate Guide

Experienced & Written By
LILACH KEREN-GRUPPER
January 2013

Copyright © 2016 Lilach Keren-Grupper. All rights reserved.

No part of this book may be reproduced or transmitted in any form or by any means, graphic, electronic, or mechanical, including photocopying, recording, taping, or by any information storage retrieval system, without the permission, in writing, of the author.

Translated from Hebrew by Sivan Gal

ISBN-13: 978-1523622924
ISBN-10: 152362292X

DISCLAIMER
This book was written by Lilach Karen Grupper, based on her personal experience of undergoing a tummy tuck surgery. It is by no means a medical guide, but a personal account of the author's experience, offering advice, tips, and guidance.

I wish you a quick recovery, a positive reading experience, a renewed sense of self-acceptance and love as well as lots and lots of fun!

Contact Information: lkgrupper@gmail.com

Table of Contents

Introduction	5
Matching Expectations	7
Before the Surgery	9
Right Before the Surgery	12
The First Meeting	15
Preparations	22
Insurance Rebates	28
The Operation	30
Waking Up from the Surgery	37
Just After	40
Night Time	46
The Following Day	48
The Release Home	51
On the Way Home	55
At Home	57
The First Shower and a Few Other Things	59
Looking After the Drains	64
A Week Later	70

Two Weeks After	72
Three Weeks After	74
Saying Goodbye to the Girdle	78
Leisure Time and Friends	81
Back to Normal	83
Final Words	85
Appendix	87
Checklist	88

INTRODUCTION

The mind, body and cognition are all aspects of a whole, which is greater than the sum of its parts. Guided by this insight, I realized that to live peacefully with all 'my parts,' I had to create an inner harmony and find a sense of self-love within; and that is exactly what I achieved by undergoing a tummy tuck surgery.

Does it sound weird? Or even shallow? Maybe. But due to the physical process I went through, I managed to develop a whole new relationship with my body which, in turn, helped me free my soul, find means of self-expression and a renewed sense of happiness.

In 1948, the term 'health' was defined as a "State of well-being, physical, mental and social; an ability to survive and adapt" and not just as a lack of disease or weakness. This term is not only used and valid today; it also serves as the basis of our collective, ongoing search for happiness.

I believe that we all possess the ability to identify, map and recognize the moment we realize we are facing something which can potentially improve our lives or the moment we realize that something really has to change. Despite the fears, the voices around me, the anxiety and what my nearest and dearest said, I felt I had to undergo this surgery, that it would serve both my physical body and my soul.

I could never have gone through it without the full support of two very precious people: my mother Liora, who ran back and forth, cooked, cared and was very proud of me, and my husband, Moti, who deeply understood me, helped me choose the right surgeon and the right timing, and made me feel I was walking down the right path.

Thanks to anyone who cheered and supported me, and last but not least, thanks to you, dear readers, for choosing to become a part of my life.

MATCHING EXPECTATIONS

Before you begin reading this guide, it is important for me to stress that, like everything in life, a tummy tuck surgery is a personal choice. Each person arrives at this decision from a particular personal, physical, mental and financial background.

We all know our body and how it has changed over the years—pregnancies, prior surgeries, weight changes, etc. It's important to be realistic about the results of the surgery.

Undoubtedly, the tummy tuck surgery will create major changes in your life. But, it's important to remember that we all begin this journey at a different point, and the surgeon (as talented as he or she may be) cannot waive the magic wand and turn us into ultra-slim models (unless we were before). The results you will see are directly related to your pre-surgery state; excess skin will be removed, your tummy will tighten, muscles will be brought closer, and you will feel like a million dollars. It's difficult to compare one post-surgery body to another, and the surgeon will match the type of operation and body sculpting, and the results will show accordingly.

I warmly recommend listening to the surgeon's advice, and pre-discuss the desired outcome.

The results of the surgery have exceeded all my expectations, and I wish you the joys of experiencing your body anew.

With love,
Lilach Keren-Grupper

BEFORE THE SURGERY

To tell you the truth, my stomach was never one to be particularly proud of or, God forbid, pierce. It was even hard to find high-cut jeans that would cover it. I always hid it. I wore tight underpants I could hardly breathe in, apologized for its shape before I gave birth, and only after three cesareans, I felt I could justify why it was as flabby, droopy and round as it was. Despite exercising steadily, I still had fat tires around it, covering and protecting it.

I'd jealously look at other mom's tummies, wondering why mine couldn't be a little more like theirs.

Some were round during pregnancy and completely flat only a month after giving birth, some were as droopy as mine, or even worse, and I would go around thinking 'how can they walk around like this?'

I started obsessing about my belly at a young age, just as my classmates began wearing tiny bikinis, or having their belly button show off under their midriff tops. I never had that. I must have skipped that phase. I was always a chubby girl; sometimes I'd lose weight and become skinny, then round again. But no matter how much I weighed, my tummy was always there. The hardest thing for me was coming to terms with it during sex. I would look at it over and over again, get angry at it, insult and denounce it. Instead of focusing on pleasuring myself and my lover, I was busy tucking it in or complaining about it. An ongoing battle: my tummy and me.

Turns out that for us women, our tummy is where we hide everything: feelings and emotions, hidden knowledge, our fertility, our ego. Some say our tummy is our first impression. In my case, all of the above is correct!

Many thoughts have traveled through my stomach, and in my search for solutions to my problem, I came across different proverbs and sayings that clarified it to me, yet again, why the tummy is so much more than just a tummy…

Here are some that stuck with me:

Butterflies in my tummy – in fact, they are in our head
Gut feeling – intuition
Bowels of the earth – deep down, inside

Tummy ache – when we're excited
Gutful – when we're angry

So, after a longstanding obsession with my belly, I decided to confront this issue once and for all and show 'it' that since it upset me for so many years, I was about to upset it back… All for a good cause though – so I could love it, reconnect with it, and feel that it's a part of me, an inseparable part of my body.

So yes…I finally went through the pregnancy and birth phase, and there isn't one woman who wouldn't agree that that's a huge relief. I lost the few extra kilograms that covered my belly as well as other body parts, started exercising four times a week and got into shape, and was finally ready to resolve my tummy issue.

I researched every option available. Electric pulses, organic drops, meditation, stomach-toning fitness equipment, Pilates classes, juice-only cleansing diet, self-awareness workshops, etc… As shallow as it may seem (I guess that's a part of me as well), none of these methods was good enough for me. I realized that if I wanted to truly get over my tummy issue, I had to take the surgical option: a tummy tuck! Wow…a dramatic decision to make, but almost secretive too, as if I was not allowed to talk about it in public; shush….my tummy tuck operation begins n-o-w!!!

RIGHT BEFORE THE SURGERY

So I'd made up my mind! Yay! Now, all that left is to learn what surgery techniques are available, hear recommendations from women who have already done it, find the right surgeon, compare prices, look at before-and-after images and start the journey.

Of course, the first point of call was the internet. I went to Google and started reading about potential surgeons; who specialized in what and where? How much experience do they have, where do they work and how commercialized they'd become. Unfortunately, the plastic surgery market is very media and celebrity-infused, and it took time to work out who was truly genuine and reliable.

It was very clear to me - I didn't want a known, famous surgeon, but a professional, reliable one.

It's not easy to find such a doctor, and as a prospective client, it was hard at the beginning to know who was just good at marketing, and who was interested in giving the most professional service throughout the process.

Since Moti, my partner, is a doctor himself, I let him guide me in the process of choosing the right doctor. He knew he wanted to go with a listed plastic surgeon, who works in one of the major hospitals as well as having a private practice. One that would be able to answer all Moti's questions, and believe me, he had lots: How many similar cases have you operated? What is the rate of infections ? How were they resolved? Would you recommend such an operation for your partner? And on and on it went...

Moti led a thorough research phase – he checked, asked, researched, found out information and gained professional knowledge on the subject matter; and together, we finally chose the surgeon that was right for me. He couldn't care less about making himself a name for operating on celebrities, and came across as deeply professional, still possessing the spark of excitement from doing what he does, and the ability to strike a real connection with us.

Another important thing to take into consideration when choosing a surgeon is that it needs to be someone you feel you can trust, completely. It is the person who will help you with one of your life's most complex issues. Trusting my surgeon was an important place to get to in the process. I felt for the first time that I was in good, reliable hands, and I could be calm about the surgery (well, as calm as one can be during this process anyway).

THE FIRST MEETING

I scheduled a consultation meeting and headed over to Tel Aviv with Moti (of course). It was a long, emotional drive; judging by my levels of excitement, I was on my way to the operation itself! We entered a fancy Tel Aviv high-rise with a swish and six super-fast elevators and headed over to the 20th floor.

As we headed out of the elevator, I sprinted to the toilet, sat down, took in a deep breath and gathered myself. I washed my hands and face, freshened up a bit from the drive, and was now ready to go into the clinic. We were welcomed by a lovely secretary who apologized for the doctor being late. "It's Ok," I answered, and we sat down in the waiting room. I was feeling very anxious and started hearing the voices in my head saying: *What do you need this for? You look great, you have an amazing family, are you losing it?* And on it went… *If I keep waiting here, I will end up running out, so I better get in quick.*

The secretary apologized again and smiled at me, trying to reassure that everything was just fine. 'Lilach, gather yourself, this is a first consultation meeting that's all.' I kept calming myself down. We finally went in, the Doctor greeted us and offered me a seat, and I, as usual, started the conversation: "I want to do a tummy tuck surgery," I said.

The doctor listened and asked: "Have you finished giving birth?"

"Sure," I answer determinedly.

"Good, let's see what we have here." I went over behind the screen to get ready: I pulled my shirt up a little bit and pulled my pants down to my knees. The doctor looked at me, examined the situation, asked me to turn around and then returned to his desk. I got dressed and went back to the room, where both he and Moti were waiting.

The doctor explained my medical condition with fairly dry, professional words: "What we have here is a looseness of the abdominal wall muscles, skin excess, and subcutaneous fat. I also found an umbilical hernia and the area you are most bothered by is called the Pinafore." He continued on to an animated clip with which he explained the surgical procedure to me:

> "I operate crossways, bring the muscles closer and tie them, remove the excess fat, stretch the loose skin and remove the excess skin so the navel is repositioned and the excess skin and fat are removed."

"Is this a tummy tuck surgery?" I asked.

"Yes," he replied.

He continued on to explain about another option called a "peripheral tummy tuck." I asked the doctor what this procedure meant, and he explained:

> "A peripheral tummy tuck includes lifting the buttocks and stretching loose back skin."

"Do I need that too?" I kept on hassling him… The doctor smiled to himself and asked:

> "Does this part of your body bother you? Because basically, you don't need anything, it's all a matter of feeling. My job is to help you with what bothers you the most so that you finish the procedure happy and content. With your back, it can go either way, so it's really up to you to make the decision. I think you'll be really happy and pleased with the normal tummy tuck surgery."

"Owww…" I breathed out heavily, I still didn't fully understand the differences between a normal operation and a peripheral one, and handed it over to Moti. "It's your turn," I said, and Moti began asking the questions he'd prepared in advance in order to understand the meaning of the procedure I was about to undergo:

> "How many cases such as this have you operated?"

"What is the post infection percentage on your operations? (I told you he is an Infectious Disease Specialist…)

"Where does the operation take place? Is it near a big hospital in case something goes wrong?"

"What are the potential complications? Which complications have you come across?"

"What are the future ramifications?"

"How long is the recovery period? And the treatment itself?"

"Would you send your wife to have this kind of operation?"

At this moment, the doctor stops, calls his wife and asks her to come into the room. A fifty-year-old woman enters the room. She is a very good-looking woman.

"Hi," she smiled at us. "I am the doctor's wife, and I also underwent the operation." "Well," I pleaded with her, "can we see?"

"Sure," she replies and immediately exposes her sculpted tummy.

"Wow," I couldn't help myself and I gasped at the sight. Moti was also amazed to see how good her tummy looked.

"Would you like to see a 'before' shot?

"Yes please," I quickly replied.

The doctor opened a folder on his computer and showed us photos of his wife's tummy as well as of other female patients.

"Are these photos taken on the day of the operation?" I asked him.

"That's right," he assured me.

"This is how they came in? With such huge bellies? How did it come off?"

"This huge tummy you are looking at is, in fact, excess belly skin and fat, and this is what I remove in the surgery."

"So I don't need to lose any weight? At the moment my BMI is ok, but I'm not skinny. Can I still do the operation?"

"The answer is yes!" the doctor said. "Of course, you have to maintain the result by entering a basic exercise regime. Drastic weight gain or pregnancies may ruin the results of the operation."

I could feel the excitement rising up in me and thought to myself, "Yay, I can solve my tummy issue right here, right now!"

"Thank you," I replied and asked Moti if he had any other questions. He didn't, and so our first meeting concluded.

A few months went by, and I felt ready for it. I scheduled a second meeting in order to decide which surgery to do – the normal or the peripheral tummy tuck. This time, I went alone.

"I want to really understand the difference between the two operations," I said to the doctor. "What effect will it have on me? How will I look with the peripheral and how will I look with the regular tummy tuck?"

The d octor was extra patient. He explained to me that the regular tummy tuck is the basis for both procedures, but the peripheral one further stretches the buttocks and the sides of the belly, not just the front. I was beginning to understand that even though I was not the classic candidate for a peripheral tummy tuck, I still wanted to go for it, despite the fact the doctor thinks that I'd be satisfied with just the regular procedure. If I was going to do this – I wanted to go the whole way. After all, it's not every day that I go under full anesthesia.

"It's your decision," he says. "You are a borderline peripheral case, which is why I am leaving it to you to make the final decision; I cannot recommend you either way."

"I understand,' I replied. "Could I speak with your wife?" I asked him.

"Sure; schedule a phone meeting with her."

I left the room feeling confused again, but deep inside me, I knew what the answer was. There's just a little bit of road to take still before I reach it wholeheartedly.

The secretary escorted me over to make the appointment for the final operation. It was scheduled for January 2013.

It's best to do the tummy tuck surgery during wintertime; when everyone is running around in the rain, you will be all snuggled up under the covers, inside a girdle. And besides, this summer you'll be wearing a bikini anyway!

The phone conversation with the surgeon's wife sealed the deal – I realized that if I didn't go for the full peripheral procedure, I would regret it later…

Moti supported me in whatever decision I made, and we were ready to go for it, all the way.

PREPARATIONS

Like any other well-planned operation, this is something you have to be prepared for well in advance, in every aspect of life:

WORK:

Inform your supervisor about the upcoming surgery and set aside a month of sick leave.

It's really important to undergo the surgery relaxed, knowing there is someone there who will take over your workload, and allowing you the calmest healing period before you go back to your normal life routine.

Make sure to take an optimal break, allowing the body and the mind quality healing time. Who knows, you may even enjoy the rest.

So... I informed my supervisor, distributed my workload around my peers, checked how many sick leave days I had in store and wished myself good luck!

HOME:

If the household chores are mainly on your shoulders…this is a great opportunity to share the load around; you will be surprised to realize how well the rest of the family members can deal with laundry, washing, cleaning chores, cooking, etc. The most important thing is that during the first two weeks after the operation you are able to rest quietly and not boss everyone around the house. Even if they don't do it exactly as you would, learn to let it go… (not an easy task).

The fridge was full, there was frozen food ready for at least two weeks, and I'd asked my relatives to make me vegetable and other light, easily digestible soups. I pre-hired a cleaner and left the other chores in Moti's hands (he even excelled at it!).

CHILDREN:

It's crucial to prepare the children for the first few weeks following the operation. Explain the process you are about to undergo to them in advance, explain that you won't be able to carry them, dress them , prepare, iron, etc. straight away.

If your children are still very young, it's really important you organize a helper in advance. The older, more sensitive children need you to prepare them for your return – you will have drains attached to your body (not a particularly thrilling sight), so best to show them images of drains and explain how they help in removing excess fluids, and that they are there to help you recover faster.[1]

I made sure not to deviate too much from the kids' usual daily routine. For example, if they had an after-school activity, I made sure they continued going in the two weeks following the operation. I made sure we had a babysitter as well as help from friends and family (this is the time to ask), especially with driving the children to their activities, etc. Our home was completely ready for allowing me the space to make my dream come true.

Hospital bag:

Just like when you're giving birth, it's important you have all your personal belongings with you so that you can feel right at home. A tummy tuck surgery includes an overnight stay in the hospital, and I

---

[1] The drains are small bottles attached to thin tubes that enter your body through the pubic area. The time it takes to remove them varies from one patient to another, in my case, it took exactly a week.

warmly recommend bringing what makes you feel cozy. For me, it was my facial crème, body lotion, make-up, favorite socks, hairbrush, toothbrush and toothpaste, a hair band (if you use one), an Ipad, cell phone and a charger. I also bought a zip-up robe, because wearing a belt could be painful around the stitches area. It's also great to bring flat sole shoes that can be easily worn (flip-flops of any kind are great).

Medicines and pharmaceuticals:

Even though you can always buy things after the surgery, it's important you have the following medical equipment at home:

An antibacterial soap for the pre-surgery shower.

Antibiotics (consult your doctor) – in case of infection

Sleeping pills – for sleepless nights (there are a few of those)

An antiseptic cream - for rubbing around the naval and the drain holes' areas.

Sterile pads – for bandaging the drain tube insertion area once the drains are out. Preferable size: 7.5 x 7.5

A long Band-Aid – for securing the pads to the drainage area once the drains have been taken out

Painkillers – for the first week after the surgery

Peglax powder – for softer excrements

Other things that may come in handy:

A thin-lined marker – for numbering the drains

Dried fruits – for softer excrements in case you haven't purchased Peglax powder. It is advised to soak the fruits in warm water and drink the water once they've cooled down.

A big pillow – for placing under your feet while asleep or resting.

An extra pillow.

Washing detergent – if you purchased one girdle, it's advised to wash it daily. While you're showering someone else can handwash and dry the girdle, so you spend the least amount of time without it.

A TV armchair – if you have one at home – great! If you don't (as was my case), it's too bad, but you can still manage without it. The most comfortable sitting/resting/sleeping position is when your legs are elevated and your back is relaxed. But, I wouldn't buy one just for the recovery period.

A plastic chair for the shower – the first showers after the operation are, well, not easy. And that's an understatement. You are likely to feel exposed without the girdle, and sometimes the blood pressure falls and you may feel you're about to faint. It's advised to shower sitting down on a chair, as well as use lukewarm water (as someone who's used to boiling water, it took some getting used to).

Lab test results:

A week prior to the surgery, you will need to pass onto your surgeon your blood test results, including chemistry, blood count, and Electrocardiogram (ECG) test results. On the day of the surgery, you will need to bring your ECG test results with you and give it to the anesthetist.

It's also advised to take the following actions prior to the operation:

> A haircut – I had my hair done a day before the surgery, it's fun to feel a sense of renewal on that front as well.
> Hair removal – it's advised to remove any hair up to a week prior to the surgery. Why a week earlier? So the skin is not irritated.
>
> Quit smoking - Smokers need to quit smoking a month prior to the operation, in order to allow the body to better heal from the procedure and let all the toxins exit the body. You can go back to smoking a month after the operation (I recommend using the surgery to quit smoking altogether).
>
> Animals at home – if you're used to sleeping with a dog, cat or any other pet (apart from your partner of course), change its location and move it to a different room.

INSURANCE REBATES

There are different rebates from different insurance agencies for different surgeries, so I can't really give you a recipe for the best, maximum insurance refund. What is important to know, though, is that the refunds (as well as the payments) are divided into three main areas -

- Hospitalization and operating room hours
- Surgeon's fee
- Girdle

It's important to get separate receipts for the three different parts, as well as something documenting the shipping delivery and the model (specifically for the girdle).

In case you are working with different insurance agencies simultaneously, it's worth investing that little bit of extra money in finding professionals who will organize the refunds. Each agency has different policies, conditions and medical reviews, so in order to exhaust all your options, I suggest loosening the rope and letting the professionals handle it.

Which is exactly what I did. I approached a professional company, which has proven to be a very good one financially. I looked for someone who used to work at an insurance agency and is deeply familiar with how these things work, as well as someone I could communicate with easily and freely. When I found the person who was right for me, I gave her my medical reviews and a full power-of-attorney, and from then on, she did all the work. She took care of the proper distribution of receipts, communicated with the different insurance agencies, spoke on the phone, sent papers and drew up professional documents pre-surgery. So all I had left to do was enjoy her professionalism and await refunds I never thought I'd get so much back. Look for someone who's reliable, professional, knows their job back to front, and is easy to communicate with. I promise you, it's a great feeling to know you're in safe hands.

The most important tip I can offer as far as insurance matters go – let the professionals do the work, it's beneficial for everyone. Also, start once you have a set date for the surgery in order to allow the both of you maximum preparation time.

THE OPERATION

It was hard to believe, but the surgery date had finally arrived. I prepared everyone around me (and myself, as much as possible). I was scheduled to be operated second and had to be at the hospital in the early hours of the morning. I had been fasting for eight hours, no food or drink of any kind (too excited to eat anyway!), and I had been tossing and turning all night long. I woke up at 5 am, and all I wanted was to do it already and be done. By the end of the day, I knew I would have been operated on, fallen in love with myself again and that I had accomplished my mission with great success! My bag was packed and ready, the girls were still asleep, and my parents arrived at our place to look after them, their eyes were swelled up with tears, but I was doing my best to ignore their anxieties and stay focused on my mission. I had taken one last shower before I got my new tummy, remembering to use the antibacterial soap. I dressed up nicely and stayed positive and in good spirits. I removed all rings, earrings and other jewelry, kissed my girls goodbye and off we went. The drive was easy, Moti was there to calm me down, and I was saying to myself: *This is it. This is my time to look after myself, and I am positive I am doing the right thing for myself.*

We arrived at the hospital five minutes late (can't escape traffic even when you leave home at 5 am!).

When we got to the hospital, we were greeted by two receptionists who were a bit blurry and confused (lucky I wasn't!). I took out the documents, which included the lab test results and the insurance policies, and ran through the full procedure with them.

It's really important to know as much as possible in advance; the insurance specialist I worked with prepared me well - I knew exactly what I was supposed to pay, I knew what was yet to be determined as far as fees go (how long the surgery would take, for example) and what the hospital had to organize with the insurance companies (for example, the night I spent at the hospital was included in my insurance policy).

We filled out all the forms, made sure everything was taken care of, handed over a credit card (just as you do in a hotel) and off we went to the operating theater. The medical staff was wearing purple gowns, and I was thinking to myself: *This is great, the hospital seems colorful, and the purple is soothing and relaxing.* There were two of us in the hospital room, adjacent toilets, a TV set, and of course, free Wi-Fi. It was time to get the iPad out, log onto Facebook, and chat away. A friend of mine who had already undergone the operation spoke with me about the amazing change I was about to go through, and the deep mental impact the surgery was going to have on my life. She tried explaining it to me, and I pretended to understand, but it's one of those things that, until you actually go through it, you can't truly understand.

An hour went by. I had been running to the toilet back and forth, which was surprising considering I'd been fasting for hours on end.

The surgeon arrived, gave me a robe, asked me to undress and leave my underwear and robe on. The only bummer is that I was right in the middle of my period (it was a major bummer). I shouldn't have been, but you know how it is, a little bit of stress and all the plans go out the window. The surgeon called us over to the preparation room; Moti was right beside me, close enough to feel me for my trembling tremble. I apologized to the surgeon about my period (he couldn't care less; after all, soon enough I was going to bleed a lot more). He was focused, relaxed and at ease, and began explaining what was about to happen from then on –

"I will be drawing on your body with a marker and take photos of your body at different angles. The photos are yours; they are a part of the procedure. I only take photos of your body, not your face."

"OK," I replied and took off my robe and underwear.

"Like most people, you're asymmetrical," the surgeon said.

He must have felt my pulse rising and up and tried to put a bit of humor in it all to help me relax. My body was showing signs of stress, anxiety, nervousness and pressure and I was shaking. But at the same time, I was trying to exude a sense of excitement and maintain a cool attitude. But I was terrified! So who was I kidding?!

"Do you think I'm crazy?" I asked the surgeon.

"That's a philosophical matter," he replied smilingly.

"Yes, but my surgery is justified right?" I implored him, in an attempt to get one last boost before he started inserting the needles into my body.

"It's a personal issue," he replied. "People used to live like this their whole lives."

"Right," I replied. "But what was the quality of the lives they lived? And were they happy with themselves?"

"This is why I said it was a philosophical matter, and why I think your surgery is justified."

I finally got him to approve of my sanity (turns out I still needed this approval).

So here I was standing with blue marker lines around my tummy area, wearing my underwear and robe again. The door opened and in entered the anesthetist, a very important man, whose job was to anesthetize me and watch me for the duration of the operation.

"Hello," he said politely and looked at me and Moti.

"Do I know you from somewhere?" he approached Moti.

"Perhaps from our army service years?" Moti suggested.

"Right! We served together for a while."

The anesthetist said smilingly; they began chit-chatting amongst themselves while I was just standing there....*Hello! I'm the one about to undergo surgery... a little bit of attention won't hurt!*

The anesthetist went through my ECG test results, asked other medical questions as well as questions regarding my weight (important information for him to have), in order to decide how much anesthetic to prescribe. He explained the process to me; I asked him to look after me, he promised and assured me that that was his job, and that's what he was there to do.

"I don't have good veins," I said. "They're hard to find," I kept going.

The anesthetist smiled (again) and said, "Well, worst case scenario, we will have to send you home." Ok, I got it, stop hassling him, everything would be just fine!

"You chose an excellent surgeon," he reassured me. "One of the best in the country."

We're heading back to the hospital room. I had to go to the toilet once more, and then a hospital orderly arrived with a wheelchair. "Please sit down," he said. For whatever reason, patients need to be wheeled into the operating room. I sat down in the chair, and couldn't believe this was actually happening. Moti got to take one photo of me and the glass doors opened; I was in the operating theater. Classical music in the background, state-of-the-art equipment, the room even seemed nicely designed. I climbed onto the bed with my arms stretched out. The anesthetist joked about sending me home again if they failed to find my veins. The medical team was ready—the surgeon, the anesthetist, a sterile nurse and an operating theater nurse.

The anesthetist tied my hand and within seconds found a good vein, into which he inserted the IV. I complemented him and felt as though I was in the best hands possible.

"I'm now going to inject you with a milk-like white liquid, you will feel a light sting in your hand, and then you'll get a bit dizzy and fall asleep."

"I already feel my hand burning, here comes the dizzy spell."

I smiled and fell into a deep, deep sleep. Sleep like I had never experienced before. As if I was not there at all and time had stopped. I had no control over what was going on, and to be frank, even though I couldn't feel anything, it was the greatest feeling ever. Perhaps surrendering full control isn't such a bad idea after all…

WAKING UP FROM THE SURGERY

I opened my eyes, shut them back, and then open again. I was somewhere between sleep and wakefulness, but mainly sleep.

"Is that it? It's all over?" I asked.

In the corner of my eye, I caught a glimpse of the anesthetist and then fall asleep again. I realize I'd done it; I'd gone through with it and come out the other end. I took a breath, and then a huge sigh of relief, filled with pride and satisfaction. *I did it!! I've been waiting for this moment for so long, it's hard to believe, but it's actually here.*

I had dreamt and fantasized about that moment for so long. I'd reached every goal I'd set for myself, I overcame all the fears, ignored background noises which had, for a while there, stopped me from going ahead with it. It was hard for me to articulate the feeling of knowing I'd gone through with it. Of achieving something so great, which for a while there seemed unattainable, and was now my new reality.

Moti came into the recovery room, caressed me confidently and whispered in my ear, "Sweetheart, you've done it," and I replied, "I'm so awesome aren't I?" He nodded in agreement, and I fell asleep again.

I woke up an hour later and was taken to the hospital room opposite the nurses' station (this operation demands close monitoring at first). I also had Moti sitting right beside me. For some reason, I was not in any pain... lucky me! I was euphoric and completely excited. Turns out, the pain comes later...But not to worry, it's not at all unbearable or unmanageable. I looked at myself, all wrapped in a girdle which went all the way from my waist to my chest. Who would've thought I could get myself into something like this? It looked like a size small girdle, and I was all squished in it like a sparkly water bottle that's been tossed around from one side to the other - once you open it, it'll splash everywhere. That's what it felt like, that the girdle was going to explode any minute, and I would pour out of it uncontrollably.

There were four drains attached to tiny bottles which were already filling up with a transparent red fluid.

"What is this?" I asked Moti, and he explained:

"These are the drains which drain out the liquids from the surgery area; there are two for the back and two for the tummy."

"Great," I said. "And how come I don't feel any pain?"

"Because you're still under the anesthetics, plus you were given painkillers towards the end of the operation. There are anesthetics inside the incisions themselves, and these will remain active for 72 hours."

On top of all that I was getting liquids and antibiotics via an IV, so all in all, it was not a great sight. My thighs were wrapped with special breathable lining pads, which helped the blood circulation. At this stage, it's definitely great NOT to be able to feel the body whatsoever.

JUST AFTER

I wanted to get up to go to the toilet, but the nurses didn't particularly approve of the brisk, opinionated patient who wanted to get out of bed three hours after a tummy tuck surgery.

"You can't get up until 8 pm," the nurse said.

"I usually get up fast; I've already had three cesareans," I bragged as if my surgical history should win me brownie points over other patients (as per usual, I'm in competition with everyone else and need to show that I'm different or stronger).

"Doesn't matter," the nurse replied despondently. "You still can't get out of bed yet."

Oh well…what am I suppose to do now? I had to go to the toilet, plus, I was on my period. Not having too many options on my hands, I tried passing the time chatting to Moti, playing on the iPad, making a few phone calls. I could see Moti needed a bit of a break, and I told him to go to the nearby shopping center to meet up with a friend. I was sharing the room with another patient, who was asleep most of the time. For the life of me, I couldn't understand how she managed to sleep; I felt high, full of adrenaline, I wanted to jump around and she was fast asleep (lucky her). At one point, she woke up, and we started chatting and sharing our experience with the process so far.

"What kind of surgery did you do?" I asked her.

"I did a tummy tuck, breast augmentation, and lip enhancement."

"Wow…you did it all at once?"

"Yes, if I'm going for it I might as well go for the whole nine yards."

And here I thought I was a hero!

"Who was your surgeon?" she asked me.

"We were operated by the same Dr, you went in before me," I replied.

"And how old are you?" I continue.

"Thirty-five, you?"

"Thirty-seven."

"How many kids?" I asked her, and she told me she has four kids. "I have three daughters," I said. The conversation continued; we talk about the reasons which led us to go for the operations, what we were like before, how long we'd planned it etc. Turns out, our needs were very similar; doesn't matter what your background is, how many children you have and where you're at in your life, we all want to feel good about our bodies and minds, they are so intrinsically interlinked.

Two hours had gone by and I still needed to go to the toilet, badly. I called the nurse again, but the answer was still no.

Moti came back feeling guilty for having left me on my own for so long. "It's all good," I said to him, "I was chatting away with my roommate here. It's good you took some time off, you'll be stuck with me for quite a while now."

My sister called and asked if she could come over to visit me. "Sure," I replied. Not half an hour went by, and my sister Nitzan arrived. At first, she was a bit shocked at the sight of the drains but was very impressed with my new figure.

The drain bottles were now half-full, and it was time to empty them out. I hassled the nurse again, this time for the drains. She emptied them out and put a sticker with a number on each one. Nizan updated me on what was going on in her life, and the hours passed by. It was 6:30 pm and I couldn't hold it anymore, I really had to go to the toilet. I really had to, but I wouldn't use the bedpan.

I called the nurse one more time and, this time, I was very decisive.

"I have to get up, and I feel that I can," I said with full confidence. The nurse wasn't happy about it, but I kept pushing it, and finally she approved my request.

"First you need to sit up in bed," she said and offered me her hand for support. I slowly rose up and sat, then lowered my legs down towards the floor and waited. Getting up for the first time after a tummy tuck operation isn't an easy task.

"Now, put your feet in the flip-flops, and carefully stand up, use me for support."

I was an excellent patient, and I did exactly what she told me to do. She followed me to the cubicle and stayed to monitor me while I took the much-awaited pee, via a special opening in the girdle. The same opening the drains went through as well as my menstrual blood. But I was so happy I finally got to do it!

"Now we go back to bed," the nurse said. With her support, I got up again and walked back to bed taking the smallest steps.

"Can I sit on the armchair?" I asked the nurse, and she agreed. She helped me sit down. Suddenly, I felt nauseous, black circles flickered around me, I couldn't breathe, and I was sweating as if I'd just finished running a full marathon.

"Moti," I called out, "I'm about to faint."

Moti lifted my legs up in the air. He said that I was pale but that fainting while sitting down is impossible. A few seconds went by, and the sweat got even more severe, the black circles were also bigger, and I could hear Moti calling a nurse over. The nurse arrived and said, "I thought you're brave." I could hear her mumble as she was pushing the armchair back to a lying position. She placed a wet, cold compress on my forehead while a second nurse checked my blood pressure.

"70/40," she said to the other nurse, "her blood pressure dropped." I could slowly feel the blood flowing again, and my face went back to its normal color.

"Did I give you a fright?" I asked Moti.

"You didn't give us a fright, but it wasn't great either to see you like this, you and your fainting feats."

As someone who suffers from low blood pressure, I am familiar with these situations, but I must admit this was a particularly severe one.

I went back to bed to keep resting, relieved that I no longer had to go to the toilet so badly.

"When will I be able to take a shower?" I asked the nurse.

"Only when you get home," she replied.

Two days after the operation. The no shower part was a bit difficult for me, but there was nothing I could do about it. Evening came, I told Moti to go home and promised myself to try and get some sleep that night.

I was so curious to see my new tummy. "Patience is a virtue," I reminded myself the sentence I always say to my daughters; it centered me and reminded me to stay positive and patient throughout this process.

NIGHT TIME

So basically, I was supposed to be really exhausted and tired. My roommate was still asleep again, and me? Wide awake! I watched TV, chatted on the phone, and felt bad for interrupting her sleep. But she was sound asleep, hardly even moved at all. *Well, what am I going to do with myself? How will I go through a whole night of this?* I started to feel pain in my abdominal area, not something I couldn't handle, but still, why should I suffer if I didn't have to? I called the nurse over and asked her for painkillers. She changed over my IV, emptied out my drains and here we went again, I was lying still in bed like a log, without being able to move or do anything. It was already 2 am and I still hadn't slept at all, as if I'd taken some kind of energy pill. *Where is all this energy coming from?* Now, when I had all the time in the world to rest, all I wanted was to run around. Crazy isn't it?! I wanted a bit of a break from my life's fast pace. I wanted to stop for a moment, give my body and soul a bit of quiet time, but now, when I had all the conditions to do exactly that, I couldn't seem to relax into it.

I gave up and asked the nurse for a sleeping pill.

And finally, I fell asleep, a peaceful, happy sleep. I still couldn't believe I was on the other side; I'd done it. It all seemed like a beautiful dream.

"Good morning," I was greeted by the morning shift nurses. I could hear them passing the information amongst themselves, updating the new nurses about my fainting feat last night and my active temperament.

"I'll be better behaved today," I tried to convince them. My roommate was still asleep. *How much can one person sleep?!* (I was totally jealous)

THE FOLLOWING DAY

Food, someone bring me food… After two full days of fasting, I was feeling the hunger alright. But all I got to eat was a low-fat yogurt and a cup of tea. "Take it slow," said the nurse, while I was dreaming of a good-sized steak…

That day, I was able to get out of bed on my own, and go to the toilet, hallelujah! What a needed, wonderful activity it is. I straighten up slowly, removed the thigh pads and confidently stood up, marching away to the much-awaited toilets. I brushed my teeth, freshened up, realized that a full shower was still a bit farfetched, but all I wanted was to wash my hair and feel at home. "Is there a towel anywhere?" I asked the nurse, and she immediately came over with a fresh white towel. Lucky I had brought my favorite shampoo, with that all too familiar smell I love so much. I turned on the tap and adjusted the temperature. I leaned over and placed my head under the water stream, and immediately felt a change in my mood. *How can such a simple task such as washing have such a deep psychological impact?* When I was done, I wrapped my hair in a white folded up towel as if I was in a fancy Spa resort. Then I then walked, hunched over, towards my bag. I took out my facial moisturizer, body lotion and hairbrush, and reveled in the feeling of feeling refreshed. The room filled up with beautiful smells, and all that was left to do was to get rid of the hospital robe and wear my own.

"We did it, we did it," I hummed the Dora tune to myself as I changed into my speckled pink robe I'd bought especially for this special occasion. Not as easy as a task as it sounds, by the way. But I handled it, even with the drains (damn those drains). I put on a new pair of socks and was now officially ready for a day of recovery, together with my sleepy roommate, who had just woken up. I urged her to wake up, and then shared my experiences from the three cesareans I had with her; the more up and active you are, the quicker and better your recovery is. She didn't seem all that enthusiastic about my active style but tried it anyway. And so we shared a morning of deep conversations about the meaning of life, stumbled over to the toilets, had our drain bottles emptied by the nurses and became acquainted with the post-surgery routine.

It was lunchtime, I had some soup and tried to rest a little bit, hoping I'd succeed this time. I managed to fall asleep, but when I woke up, the pain was slightly more intense. Still completely manageable, though. My mom came over for a visit; she took one look at me and it was clear she was dissatisfied with the decision I'd made.

"Mom, it's mine! It's my decision, my body. I owed it to myself."

Some people may disapprove of your decision, or won't understand it. And you know what? Even if some people think I'm crazy, so what?! I'm so happy with the decision I made, and with how I did it, every step of the way. My husband completely supported me, and everyone else, really, it's just too bad!

No one can fully know another person's soul, or what is good for someone else like we know ourselves. Something can seem completely wrong to one person, but can be the best thing in the world for someone else. Reconnecting with myself again is a major upgrade to my life, not just to my appearance. I find myself feeling more whole than I have ever been (despite the cuts and the stitches), and happier than I've ever been (despite the pain). Happy for my ability to go through with something I have wanted and waited for, for so long.

THE RELEASE HOME

It was late afternoon; the surgeon came to release us to go home! I couldn't wait to get back, to my daughters, my things; even though the hospital stay itself was very pleasant, there's no place like home.

My roommate had received instructions about her release, and now it was my turn; he asked how I was doing, explained the process of the surgery and what he did, and said he was very pleased with the results (he'd better be!).

"I just want to see my new tummy," I urged him.

I lay in bed; he closed off the screen and explained to me what I would need to do at home –

"The drainage bottles need to be emptied out when the fluids reach 20ml. In the beginning, you will empty it every eight hours, and after about two days, it will change to every twelve hours. You will need to write the exact amount of fluids in each drain bottle, and then hang it back up on the girdle."

"Sounds pretty easy and manageable," I said.

"You can take the first shower tomorrow," he continued, "seated on a chair and supervised. But we'll talk about it over the phone later. It's very important to take your painkillers every four hours; you shouldn't suffer through it."

I listened to him intently but didn't really understand what he was talking about, because up until then, the pain really wasn't so bad. But I was starting to sense that the hard part was yet to come.

He opened the girdle. "The girdle is made of hooks, and what seals it hermetically is a zipper that is placed above the hooks." He quickly unzipped the girdle and said, "Say hello to your new naval."

"Wow," I was completely exalted. "It's incredible! Is this really my new tummy?"

I was reacquainted with my own abdominal area, and it already felt like love at first sight. I was in love with it, and it looked back at me, yearningly, as if it had finally managed to please me, after years of constant battle.

"The swelling will decrease as your healing progresses," the surgeon said, and I thought to myself: *What swelling? If this is swollen, it means my tummy will be even flatter and smoother than this!* I was elated.

"Thanks so much," I replied.

"We'll be in touch tomorrow, and good luck," he said and left.

My mom returned to the room, the surgeon shook her hand and moved on to the next patient. "That's it, Mom, we can go and sign off on the release documents, let's call the nurse."

The nurse came over, took out the IV and sent me to the reception to finalize the bill. I stumbled over towards the reception area, supported by my mom. It somehow felt like a long way from my room, even though when we got here, it didn't seem that far at all. I was finally at the reception desk after getting lost on the way twice (that's what happens when every step is a major task). My mom and I waited for the couple that was already there to finish so we could sit down and finalize everything, but they just keep on sitting there, all peaceful and calm.

"Excuse me," I approached them gently with the final shreds of courtesy I still had left in me before it dissipated.

"I've just had an operation and I need to finish things off at the reception."

The couple looked at me when suddenly they realized how pale I was and saw the drains attached to the girdle. They got up at once and offered us their chairs. "Thanks," I said while in pain, and asked the secretary to take out my paperwork.

It was the same paperwork from yesterday, only this time it was filled with lots of details, including billable operating theater hours. She took me through all the costs; I verified everything, but

I made sure to mention that the overnight stay costs were covered by my private insurance, since I'd had my umbilical hernia mended (again, I was well prepared in advance for this). She made a few phone calls, and everything was sorted.

Home…I just want to get home. I went back to my room, collected whatever stuff I had left there, passed the reception letter to the nurses, said farewell to my roommate, and again, helped by my mother, I stumbled over to the lift which took us through the shopping center down to the car park.

An Israeli song by the name of "Long Road" was playing at the mall, and I was thinking to myself that it was a lovely coincidence. It had been a long road for me, but here I was, on the other side. The same singer has another song which I love, where she says to other women 'Do what you love doing / Anything you want / Do whatever makes you happy….'"

Who, if not us, is in charge of our external and internal happiness?

I felt a real sense of victory.

ON THE WAY HOME

My mom's car was parked close to the escalators. They too seemed a bit mission impossible. My mom held me as I climbed onto the escalator. I was a bit shaky when the moment came to get off the stairs. Every trivial action had become a challenging task. Definitely a good lesson for life – appreciate what you have. I kept reminding myself that this was a temporary condition and that soon enough I'd be able to climb the stairs in a bikini. "How do I get into the car?" I asked my mom (as if she should know). She opened the car door; I grabbed hold of the top handle, moaning and groaning my way into the car. Now all that was left was to adjust the seat to the best position, for me, it was half lying down. Once I was comfortable, we got on the road. The road home seemed longer than ever. The rain drizzled out the window, and Haifa seemed so far from Tel Aviv.

It was dark and the traffic was heavy. I could feel every bump on the road, every little rock. After a while, I could see Haifa's lights in the distance; soon we'd be home.

I had never been so happy to see our driveway. "Here I come baby," I started talking to the driveway as if it could hear me. My mom parked carefully, and then helped me get out of the car. I climbed down the stairs; couldn't wait for a warm, fuzzy hug from my daughters.

AT HOME

"Mom…..!" they all run towards me together.

"Easy now, don't jump on me. I'm in pain and hunched over.

"What have they done to you," my 9-year-old daughter asked me.

"Are you going to be ok?" asked the 6-year-old, and the youngest one, who's only 3 said, "Mommy you've got bottles dangling off your body."

I was trying hard not to laugh and quickly explained to them that I'm ok, I'm in a bit of pain after the operation but happier than ever.

"The bottles extract the unnecessary fluids out of my body, so my tummy doesn't bloat out," I explained.

Sahar, my eldest, quickly understood what was going on and offered her help. "We'll behave," she promised (let's see how long this one lasts).

"We'll help you," my middle one said while their younger sister was already off asking Moti for whatever she needed. I headed over to our bedroom, and the first thing I did was change to cozy, comfortable clothes. This was when Moti became my personal assistant and helped me do just about anything – get up, put on socks, get dressed, go to the toilet, and many other daily routine actions.

The girls were getting used to my temporary disability and tried (as much as they could) to be considerate. It was nighttime, so I carefully crawled into bed, and regretted not having bought an adjustable bed… Moti brought a large pillow and rested it under my feet, and another one for my head; this turned out to be the most comfortable position under the circumstances.

I couldn't sleep again; the pain started, like an electric shockwave, in localized pulses. Moti got me a painkiller, which was a derivative of morphine. It's the best thing he could have given me at the time. I managed to sleep for a little while and woke up to a new morning.

Today is shower day! I was so happy that I almost forgot I hadn't had any poop over the past few days. The surgeon's wife called to see how I was doing and to guide me before my first shower. Turns out the much-awaited shower was not that easy a task and demanded specific preparations.

THE FIRST SHOWER AND A FEW OTHER THINGS

The orders I received for the first shower were very specific, and I made sure to follow them diligently:

An hour before taking the shower I needed to take a painkiller. Why an hour before? So the painkiller reaches its maximum effect while I shower.

Place a plastic chair in the shower, a foot stool, towels, antiseptic cream, q-tips with which you rub the antiseptic cream, natural body cream, comfortable clothes (socks, underwear, bra, pants, shirt), and most importantly – have someone there to help you with it all.

Moti and I were getting ready; we had planned it for the late hours of the morning while the girls were already at school and pre-school, and everything was ready.

I laid in bed, and Moti took off the girdle. He carefully unzipped the side zippers, and unhooked the hooks one after the other. I was sure this was the moment I would spill out of the girdle, but surprisingly enough, there was nothing to spill out… Slowly but surely Moti peeled off my second skin (the girdle), and while he did that I held onto the drains and pulled them through the girdle hole. At the beginning, we tried passing the drains together, but this system didn't prove fruitful – sometimes taking shortcuts only elongates our way – so instead, I recommend pulling them through in pairs or one by one.

Body odor mixed with clotted blood filled the air (luckily, Moti didn't choke)

"We have to wash it, quickly," I said, but Moti suggested we do it after I take the shower.

I looked at my tummy – it was still swollen from the trauma of the surgery, but it looked gorgeous! With all the contusions, stitches, threads, Band-Aid s and bruises decorating it, I still imagined myself walking around with a tight pair of pants, normal underpants, g-string, bikini…

Moti gave me his hand for support and said "Let's do it, off to the shower." He knew how long I had waited for this. I walked in carefully, Moti washed me with lukewarm water, and I was basking in the pleasure of this much-awaited moment. I hummed songs to myself while he shampooed my head and body. I could feel myself getting addicted to the feeling of the water and the soap on my body.

After about half an hour of pure pleasure, I decided it was time to get out. Moti placed a warm towel over my head and my body, wiped off my feet (I couldn't bend down), I held the drains and headed out towards the chair outside the shower, which was waiting for me all wrapped with clean, warm towels. I sat down to catch my breath. It was only a shower but I felt as if I'd just completed an extreme mountain bike challenge (and I don't even ride). The black circles returned, I'm pale again.

"Moti, I'm fainting" I called out, and this is when the stool came into the picture. Moti brought over the stool, lifted my feet up and cooled me down with a wet, cold cloth. "Can't stand these fainting feats," I mumbled as Moti put me back to bed.

"It's best you lie down with your feet up" he said, and I complied.

Within seconds, I was back to normal and joking about the whole thing.

"Let's wash this girdle before the neighbors come looking for a dead body," I said and Moti helped me up.

Since I only bought the one girdle (which I now regretted), I had to wash and dry the one I had just taken off as quickly as possible. A little bit of detergent and lukewarm water will do the trick. Moti removed the straps off the girdle (same as with bra straps), rubbed it in all the right places, and every now and then let me smell it, until I was completely satisfied with the smell. Now, the girdle needed to be dried. In this case, it was crucial to have a drier. We tried drying it out with a hair-drier, towel heater, but nothing beats the drier. (I suggest wrapping the girdle in a towel although they separate in the drier and put it in the drier for about 15-20 minutes on a cool-drying program). Meanwhile, Moti rubbed the antiseptic cream on my abdominal area, as well as the drain areas, using the q-tips.

Once I'd finished rubbing natural oil, dried off completely and covered the new holes with the antiseptic cream, the girdle was ready for re-use. I had no idea how to put that thing back on. "Perhaps lying down?" I suggested, and we decided to give it a try. We laid the girdle open on the bed, and I rolled myself onto it in the right position. We passed the drains through the girdle hole, then zipped up the right-hand side zipper, and then moved onto the hooks. Then, we moved onto the left-hand side. If you ever wondered what cooperation means, well, this is it. My legs were already wrapped in, but my waist area refused to be squashed back in for some reason. I pulled the two sides of the girdle closer together and Moti zipped it up, and I closed off the hooks. Slowly but surely, my body fit back into the girdle.

"This was tough," Moti said.

"Mission impossible," I added. But not to worry, it gets better, and a week later, I was already doing it completely by myself.

Time to get dressed. I put on my underpants, on top of the girdle, then pants, I hooked up the damn drains and then a bra and a shirt, and I was ready. The bottles needed to be emptied out, but the stickers had gotten wet in the shower and there were no numbers on them anymore. This is where the marker came into the picture. I wrote a number on each bottle, and wrote down the amount of fluids in each drain bottle in a table I'd prepared earlier.

I was exhausted after the shower, and finally felt like I needed to rest. I got into my cushiony bed and thankfully managed to fall sleep.

Did I mention I hadn't once pooped since the surgery? So while we're on the topic, there is a reason that I suggest preparing Peglax powder or having dried fruits at home. One tablespoon of Peglax helps smooth down the stools (believe me, you don't want to know how painful it is to try and poop after the surgery). Within twenty-four hours, the issue was resolved and I was back on track.

LOOKING AFTER THE DRAINS

If there is one thing that's burdensome about this operation, it's the drains. Whether you come out of the operation theater with two or four drainage bottles, they're an annoying nuisance. But they do the work.

It's important to remember that the drainage holes have an extremely important role in the process, and they deserve every respect. Despite how frustrated I was with them throughout the process, I tried to remind myself of the final goal, but in all honesty, they're a real hassle.

You need to write down numbers on each drain bottle – preferably with a marker.

You need to be diligent about writing down the amount of fluids in each bottle in the table you prepared for it.

The maximum amount of fluids for emptying out is 20ml, so if one drain bottle reaches that amount, empty all of them. You need to create a vacuum in the bottles after emptying them out.

After the shower, you need to rub the antiseptic cream around the drainage holes, using a q-tip.

If one of the drain holes is bleeding due to pulling, dressing up or any other movement, you need to stop the blood, rub the antiseptic cream and report to your doctor.

A high-protein, low-carb diet is advised (always) – it lowers the amount of fluids in the body.

When do you take the drains out? When you notice that in a 24-hour collection cycle there's less than 20ml of fluids collected in each drain bottle.

Without a doubt, the drainage bottles made my life harder. They hurt, annoyed, burned and filled up so much every day, that it took a week until I could actually take them out. Every day that went by, I was so sure they're going to be taken out, but much to my dismay, the answer was negative. Luckily, the weather was so bad that it was impossible to get to Tel Aviv anyway, so there was some justification for staying with them for that long.

It had been a week since the operation, and the bottles were still filling up so much every day I was starting to lose patience. My right leg was hurting (turned out one of the tubes was pushing against a nerve), I was underslept, and I wanted them out, fast.

I was speaking with the surgeon's wife, who tried to calm me down every day, but this time, she too gave up and called me into the clinic.

I amazed myself with a sudden wave of motivation – I got myself ready, put on makeup, organized a babysitter, got Moti to come back from work and off we went back to the clinic in Tel Aviv. But not before I took a strong painkiller for the journey ahead.

Despite the pain in my right leg, the lack of sleep and how impatient I'd become, I marched into the clinic like a panther. I didn't come in with any expectations, though. Which is why I was so surprised when she said to me:

"Today we take out the drains."

"What? Who? Are you sure?" I asked.

"Yes," she replied. "What you have here looks extractable."

I must've been the happiest woman in the world and more patient than ever to wait my turn. There were other women in the corridor waiting their turn and others who were there for their pre-surgery consultation.

"Easy peasy," I said to one of them, again trying to prove to the world that I'm a superhero, that nothing's too tough for me, forgetting that up until a moment ago, I was a nervous wreck. In front of me in line was a woman who went in to take her drains out. She came back without them.

"Does it hurt?" I asked her.

"Not too bad. It's quick, and the feeling afterward is worth it all," she said smilingly.

It was my turn. I went into the doctor's room, he welcomed me, and I asked for his opinion, for the last time, about getting the drains out.

"I want you to tell me it's ok," I said and he replied without hesitation:

"It's ok."

"Then let's do it!"

He cleared off the patient bed, I took off my pants and underwear and he explained:

"I am going to arrange the drains one next to the other and I will tell you when I'm about to take them out."

"No, no, don't tell me, I prefer not to know," I replied and covered my eyes with my hands so I couldn't see him doing it.

"Ouch…it's burning, really burning!" I screamed out and then it all subsided.

In one second, the intrusive pain was gone and the drains were out.

"You don't want to know what came out of your body," Moti said while looking at me, both agonizing and cheerful at the same time.

"Show me," I asked the surgeon, and he pulled out of the bin a very, very long tube, with a serrated edge at the tip.

"There is not a chance in hell this was inside my body," I was amazed and horrified at the same time.

"Lucky you took all of them out at once, otherwise I don't think I'd have been able to go on with it."

The surgeon pulled out a bottle of ethanol and poured it over the holes, and if I hadn't fainted so far this was probably a good moment for it!

"Are you crazy?!" I yelled out. "Have you decided to finish me off completely?"

The pain has a strong burning sensation as if someone had thrown acid on me and lit me on fire. But it passed within minutes, and the joy of having the drains removed was far greater than the pain; much like birth, I said it already didn't I?

The surgeon gave us final instructions for the treatment of the drainage holes and then did it once himself to show us how it works: "After a shower, the area needs to be dried out and once it's dry, rub the antiseptic cream on the holes which are still open. Then place a pad over it and stick it with a long Band-Aid strip, until the holes stop extracting any fluids, and that's it. Easy to handle."

"We have to celebrate this moment," Moti said.

He suggested that since we were in a euphoric mode and in Tel Aviv, we should celebrate it in a feast. The surgeon's wife recommended a nearby restaurant and we headed over there, with an incredible feeling of freedom, as if we'd just been released from jail. There was still a little bit of pain but it's negligible in comparison to how it was before the drains were removed. We were completely high, eating, drinking, laughing and taking photos, with lots of people around us. It was one of the most beautiful moments in the whole process. I wouldn't pass any of it up, despite the difficulties preceding.

A WEEK LATER

Life was much easier without the drains. The pain was nearly all gone and I was almost able to stand up straight. I slept at night, was awake and vital during the day, and began writing this guide for you. Trying to convey, in words and images from my world, the sensations, thoughts and feelings I experienced during the process and afterward, hopefully I succeeded.

I was able to shower by myself without fainting; I washed the girdle by myself before I washed so it was ready when I got out. I wore it more easily, and it seemed as if it was molded to my shape.

The household chores I had delegated to everyone else were slowly coming back my way – cooking for the girls, doing the washing, etc. I hummed a favorite song while looking at my new tummy. I loved it so much. I started walking naked in front of the mirror with my head up high, taking photos from every angle (can't even remember the last time I took a photo of it, I always tried hiding it). Even with the Band-Aid s still covering the scar, it looked great. 'In love with my new tummy, thank you, thank you, thank you,' I sent an SMS to the surgeon's wife. I was starting to enjoy my sick leave, and called my family doctor, I promised to show her the results.

When I arrived, she greeted me benevolently and asked if she could take a look. I didn't even wait for her to finish the question, and already I was peeling off the girdle and showing off my new tummy.

"Wow," she was thrilled. "Well done on the result, and well done for going ahead with it, there's no reason for you to walk around with a sloppy tummy at your age."

"Really? You think I made the right decision?" Again, I was looking for external approval of my decision.

"Sure you have! Without a doubt! Now you have a tummy of a 16-year-old, there's no reason to walk around with anything that upsets or disturbs us," she replied.

"Thanks so much," I said and took the opportunity to ask for more antiseptic cream, which I was plowing through at a phenomenal rate. I left her room, walked two flights of stairs easily and walked back home (about a ten-minute walk in my current state).

TWO WEEKS AFTER

I could now safely say that the hard part was now behind us and life was getting back on track. I managed to sleep on my side, with no painkillers, and even on my tummy, without extra pillows I could shower on my own... I got out of bed easily, prepared food, did the laundry, but made sure not to carry my youngest daughter or any grocery bags. I still had to be careful and look after myself. Despite the desire to go and run a marathon, I settled for a few shoulder exercises and short walks around the block.

Sex was back too, only carefully. At this point, you can do almost anything, even with the girdle (and may I remind you there's a special hole in the right place for it).

I found driving again a bit stressful at first, but after the first two drives, the fears were gone and I was back to being the taxi driver I used to be –

driving the kids from one place to another, but… when I didn't feel like doing it, I could still use the "I'm a bit tired and need to rest excuse."

It was time to pamper myself with a neck and shoulder massage to help release all the tension that got caught up in the area due to my new sleeping positions. I still recommend to take the time and not run straight back to work (they'll wait for you for another week), use the time for uplifting activities such as shopping, especially now, when your pants size will have dropped. You can add shirts and of course, normal people's underwear, not the shaper style.

Bending down was still a little bit hard, so please - don't overdo it. There's something nice about letting other people lift things for you, and if you wish to put a bit of nail polish on your feet, make sure to use the stool.

THREE WEEKS AFTER

Another medical review. I was getting ready to leave the house, wearing a tight burgundy lattice dress, a bag on my shoulder and oh... I nearly forgot the garbage bag waiting by the door (we have a habit at home that whoever leaves, takes out the bag with them). I grabbed the bag in one hand and my handbag in the other, marching towards the large garbage disposal container. I opened it using the foot handle and bang, the garbage, and my cell phone dove in together, right into the nearly empty bin.

Oh no... What am I going to do? I could hear the phone ringing from inside the bin but I couldn't answer it. I tried to get creative, turning the bin in every direction possible. I definitely couldn't turn it upside down, and definitely not in my current state. I dragged the bin over to our driveway, climbed over the water meters, from there onto a low pole, which no one ever knows what it's doing there, and there I was, inside the bin, with the cell in my hand! Had someone seen me jumping into a green rubbish bin, after a tummy tuck surgery, they would've thought I was out of my mind. *Ok, so what now?* Good for me for getting into the bin, but I also needed to get out of it. I had a train to catch and time was of the essence. I decided to call my mom and explain my grim situation. Within seconds, Mom came over, with a huge smile on her face. The sight of me stuck inside the bin was definitely a very funny one. I had no idea how, but I'd somehow managed to overcome the difficulty of jumping out of the bin onto the cement pole, then onto the water meters, and finally back to the ground. Surely you'd agree that if I went in and out of a bin, I was on track towards full recovery…

I just made it in time for the train, made my way carefully through the crowd, and together with my mom and a good friend, was on my way back to the clinic. Still strapped inside the girdle, which was beginning to feel like a protective shield, I was nearly as excited as I was before the surgery itself. *What's going on Lilach?* I started talking to myself in my head. *You've gone through it, it's done*, I could barely contain the happiness and excitement that was bubbling up in me. As if I was about to face the final test, and the surgeon was the teacher.

We got to the fancy building; the waiting room was full of women checking each other out. The desire to ask each and every one what surgery she did undermines every social etiquette rule I'd ever known. It took us only a few seconds to know which surgery each one of us had done, even before we knew each other's names. The conversation made us all chirpy, and I have to share with you that each and every woman who was there reported a positive change in her life.

It was my turn! I went into the surgeon's room, took off the girdle and showed off the result. "We can remove the Band-Aid s," he said and pulled them off, then he cut a few stitches that emerged from the scar that was now absorbing into my skin. One or two of the stitches were bleeding, he gave me light pads and the girdle went back up.

"The scar looks great, the tummy is nice and stretched. One more week and you'll be able to get back to moderate walking exercises."

"I have one more question – can I take the girdle off every now and then? It mainly bothers me at night," I asked hesitantly.

"You can take the girdle off at night, one more week and you'll be able to take it off altogether," he replied and I got excited.

One night of sleeping without it meant quality sleep, which I hadn't had in a very long time.

"Your next review is in a month's time; you may not need the silicon straps," he added. "The silicon straps are used to flatten the scar once it's healed completely, but we'll see about that later on."

"Thanks," I replied excitedly, warmly shook his hand and headed out to the corridor.

"Alright, I deserve a bit of shopping time!" I said to my mom and sister who had just joined us and my friend.

We strolled along Eben Gabirol Street; designer shops, sun, and me! I tried on clothes (over the girdle), and everything pretty much fit and sat beautifully on my tummy. I bought a few things (expensive but worth it), and I was high as a kite.

We kept strolling around, sat in a restaurant, shopped and enjoyed the moment. This was one of best moments I had during the recovery period.

SAYING GOODBYE TO THE GIRDLE

I slept without the girdle for the first time tonight. I felt free, but at the same time vulnerable, weak and more exposed than ever. What was it in the girdle that protected me? Like an armor enveloping my body, covering it against the dangers of the outside world. I took off this protective shield I'd become so accustomed to and got into bed. At first, I found a comfortable position. But then settled for laying half on my side and half on my back, and fell into deep sleep.

When I got up, I went straight to the girdle; it looked as though it missed me too, and we became one again. I took a deep breath and squeezed myself into it. I was feeling all bundled up again, and it was extremely comfortable and really uncomfortable at the same time. A bit absurd isn't it?

I realized that saying goodbye to the girdle wasn't going to be that easy; it needed time and preparation. So I decided to plan a gradual farewell program so that both of us felt we'd been given the right amount of time to get used to the upcoming separation. I continued to wear it during the day, and at night we parted ways, it went to be washed and dried, and I went about my business. This way, after a month and a half of being completely inseparable, we both felt confident we could manage on our own. But still, I took the girdle everywhere with me, it was in my bag waiting for me in case I felt too vulnerable or exposed and needed its protection again. I did that for as long as I saw fit, until I didn't feel like I needed it anymore.

Dear girdle,

This is an opportunity to thank you for the support and protection you've given me, day and night. You never left me, you were always there, enveloping and squeezing at the same time. You protected me internally and externally, and you taught me the meaning of absurd. I could never go through this process as successfully as I did, without you.

Now, a month and a half after the operation I feel that it's time for me to put you back in the drawer, and move on (you deserve some rest too). I am off to a new and fascinating path, and I know I'll miss you and if I ever feel your absence, I can always approach you and you'll be there for me.

With great appreciation and yours truly,
Lilach

LEISURE TIME AND FRIENDS

In the first couple of weeks after the operation, I discovered an easy way to pass the time. The position that was the most convenient for me was on a good quality office chair in front of the computer, so instead of watching TV or sleeping, I discovered shopping on Amazon, eBay, and other such quality websites.

Want to know what I bought? Seven pairs of shoes, four watches, two books, three handbags and still going strong. No doubt, an empowering experience in its own right.

On top of that, friends who were curious to see the results came over, mainly to hear about the process and understand what I'd been through and was still going through.

Here are some of the responses I've received so far –

"I want to do it too."

"How much did it cost?"

"Not too expensive at all."

"Wow… but I need to lose weight first."

"Amazing!"

"Champion."

"Everything hurts?"

"You look great."

"You gave me motivation to do it too."

"What's the surgeon's phone number?"

Well, I definitely managed to create a little storm amongst my friends, relatives, and acquaintances.

BACK TO NORMAL

A month had passed since the operation. I felt like my body was in need of some serious movement other than walking from the bedroom to the computer, kitchen or outside the house.

I felt fully energized towards this next phase of – going back to normal.

Sounds so dramatic, as if some tragedy happened and I was finding my way back from it. In this case, going back to normal meant that very soon this whole thing would be behind me, after a very long time.

Sure, it made me very happy but, at the same time it was a bit hard to let go of occupying myself with it – before, during and after the operation, it was a bit like being the center of attention for a while.

I was getting myself ready for a moderate beach walk. Activewear (size S), new sports shoes I'd just purchased on Amazon, a backpack, bottle of water, cell phone and shades; I was going for a walk.

Wintery sunrays caressed my face, there was a cool breeze around and I was walking around with a huge smile on my face. *It's so good to know how to enjoy the smallest things in life*, I think to myself. Happiness itself is in my hands (or in my new tummy), and all I have left is to hug it and ask it to stay for a little while longer. I marched along the long promenade and enjoyed every step. A group of surfers went into the water to catch some waves and I enjoyed seeing them taking advantage of what the day had to offer. I started walking a little faster and felt my energy rise up. When I finished the walk, I was left with a feeling of wanting more; to walk more, smell more, breathe more, feel like I am taking in everything life has to offer, in one big breath.

The following day, I did exactly the same, and slowly but surely, I was regaining a sense of control over my body and mind again. I was doing it at the pace that was right for me, gradually, and enjoying my ability to be in tune with what I could and couldn't do each day. I took small mental and physical steps every day, and rehabilitated myself, at the pace that was right for me.

FINAL WORDS

What can I say… one of the best decisions I've ever taken.

The sense of self-acceptance I enjoy, the happiness I experience with my partner, all of this thanks to one single operation.

All I can say is that only we know what's right for us, what suits us, and when to do what we need to do.

I am finishing writing this guide with one personal, authentic message; listen to yourself, to your body and your soul, take care of your own happiness in every way you can (no one else will). No matter what path you choose to take, and what changes you decide to make (if at all), in whatever course of life – the road you will take to achieve your desired goal is the process through which you will develop, grow and learn, and give yourself the biggest gift of all – the gift of self-fulfillment.

There is much more at stake than a flat tummy. I guarantee you everyone around you will reap the rewards of your process – your partner, children, close family, work and most of all, you yourself.

When you're happy, everyone around you is too.

Appendix

A fluids-extraction follow-up table

DAY	TIME	DRAIN 1	DRAIN 2	DRAIN 3	DRAIN 4
SUN					
SUN					
MON					
MON					
TUES					
TUES					
WED					
WED					
THURS					
THURS					
FRI					
FRI					
SAT					
SAT					

CHECKLIST

Pharmaceuticals:

Dermax – antibacterial soap for the pre-surgery shower

Antibiotics (doctor's prescription) – in case of infection

Sleeping pills – for sleepless nights or trouble sleeping

Antiseptic cream – for rubbing around the naval area and drainage holes

Sterile pads – for bandaging the drainage holes after removing the drain tubes Preferable size: 7.5 x 7.5

Lost paper band aid – for attaching the sterile pads

Painkillers – for the first week only

Peglax – for softer stools

Personal items:

Facial cream

Body lotion

Makeup

Socks

Hairbrush

Toothpaste and toothbrush

Hair-band

iPad

Cell phone and charger

zip up robe

Comfortable flat shoes (flip-flops)

Recommended items:

A thin marker – for marking numbers on the drain bottles

Dried fruits – for helping to smooth excrements

A large foot pillow

An extra cushion – for naps

Hand wash laundry detergent – for the girdle

A TV armchair if you have one

A plastic chair for the shower – the first showers are taken while seated

Lab tests:

Chemistry

Blood count

ECG

Pre-surgery recommendations:

A hair cut

Hair removal – a week prior to the surgery

Quit smoking – advised a month prior to the surgery to allow the body maximum healing

Pets – if you have pets at home and you are used to sleeping with them, change the pet's location to another room

Printed in Great Britain
by Amazon